The Green Beauty Revolution: Unleashing the Power of Natural Skincare

Linda

Copyright © [2023]

Title: The Green Beauty Revolution: Unleashing the Power of Natural Skincare
Author's: Linda

All rights reserved. No part of this publication may be reproduced, stored in a retrieval system, or transmitted in any form or by any means, electronic, mechanical, photocopying, recording, or otherwise, without the prior written permission of the publisher or author, except in the case of brief quotations embodied in critical reviews and certain other non-commercial uses permitted by copyright law.

This book was printed and published by [Publisher's: **Linda**] in [2023]

ISBN:

TABLE OF CONTENT

Chapter 1: Introduction to Natural Skincare   07

The Rise of Natural and Organic Skincare

The Benefits of Natural Skincare Products

Understanding the Green Beauty Revolution

Chapter 2: The Science Behind Natural Skincare   13

The Harmful Effects of Chemicals in Skincare Products

Exploring the Power of Natural Ingredients

How Natural Skincare Works with Your Skin

Chapter 3: Building Your Natural Skincare Routine   19

Assessing Your Skin Type and Concerns

Cleansing: The Foundation of Natural Skincare

Nourishing Your Skin with Natural Moisturizers

Targeted Treatments for Common Skin Issues

Chapter 4: DIY Natural Skincare Recipes 27

The Benefits of Making Your Own Skincare Products

Essential Oils for Skincare

Homemade Facial Cleansers and Exfoliators

DIY Face Masks and Serums

Chapter 5: Shopping for Natural Skincare Products 35

Understanding Labels: Decoding Green Beauty Jargon

Choosing the Right Brands and Ingredients

Where to Buy Natural Skincare Products

Evaluating Product Claims and Certifications

Chapter 6: Overcoming Challenges in the Green Beauty Journey 43

Dealing with Transitioning Periods

Addressing the Myth of Natural Skincare Inefficiency

Overcoming Price and Accessibility Concerns

Sustainable Packaging and Eco-Friendly Practices

Chapter 7: The Future of Natural Skincare 51

Innovations in Natural Skincare Technology

The Role of Science and Research in Green Beauty

Advocating for Transparency and Regulation in the Industry

Embracing a Holistic Approach to Natural Beauty

Chapter 8: Inspiring Success Stories in Natural Skincare 59

Entrepreneurs and Brands Leading the Green Beauty Revolution

Real-Life Transformations with Natural Skincare

Celebrity Endorsements and Influencers in the Natural Beauty Space

Global Initiatives and Organizations Supporting Natural Skincare

Chapter 9: FAQs and Common Misconceptions about Natural Skincare 68

Is Natural Skincare Suitable for All Skin Types?

Can Natural Skincare Treat Serious Skin Conditions?

Debunking Myths: Natural Skincare vs. Traditional Skincare

Addressing Safety Concerns and Regulatory Issues

Chapter 10: Embracing the Green Beauty Revolution 76

Incorporating Natural Skincare into Your Lifestyle

Taking Steps Towards a More Sustainable Beauty Routine

Spreading Awareness and Inspiring Others

The Power of Natural Skincare in Transforming Lives

Conclusion: Empowering Yourself with Natural Skincare 86

Chapter 1: Introduction to Natural Skincare

The Rise of Natural and Organic Skincare

In recent years, there has been a noticeable shift in the beauty industry towards natural and organic skincare products. People from all walks of life are becoming increasingly aware of the harmful chemicals and synthetic ingredients that are commonly found in conventional skincare products. As a result, a green beauty revolution is taking place, unleashing the power of natural skincare and transforming the way we care for our skin.

What exactly is natural and organic skincare? Simply put, it refers to products that are made with ingredients derived from nature, such as plant extracts, essential oils, and minerals. These products are free from harsh chemicals, artificial fragrances, and synthetic additives that can irritate the skin and cause long-term damage.

One of the main reasons for the rise in popularity of natural and organic skincare is the growing concern for our health and well-being. Consumers have become more conscious of the potential risks associated with using products that contain harmful ingredients. They are now seeking safer alternatives that not only nourish and protect their skin but also contribute to their overall health.

Another driving force behind this revolution is the increasing awareness of our impact on the environment. Conventional skincare products often contain ingredients that are harmful to the ecosystem, as well as being produced through unsustainable practices. By switching to natural and organic skincare, we can reduce our carbon footprint and support brands that prioritize sustainability and ethical sourcing.

Furthermore, natural and organic skincare products are known for their effectiveness. Many of these products harness the power of nature to address specific skin concerns, such as dryness, acne, or aging. Plant-based ingredients are rich in antioxidants, vitamins, and minerals that promote healthy skin and can deliver noticeable results without the need for harsh chemicals or invasive procedures.

The rise of natural and organic skincare has also led to a surge in innovation within the industry. As demand grows, more brands are investing in research and development to create high-quality products that meet the needs of a diverse range of skin types and concerns. This means that there are now more options than ever before for individuals to find the perfect skincare routine that suits their unique needs.

In conclusion, the rise of natural and organic skincare is a positive and transformative trend in the beauty industry. It offers a safer and more sustainable alternative to conventional skincare products, while also delivering effective results. By embracing this green beauty revolution, we can not only care for our skin but also contribute to a healthier planet for future generations.

The Benefits of Natural Skincare Products

In today's fast-paced and highly polluted world, taking care of our skin has become more important than ever. Our skin is the largest organ in our body, and it serves as a protective barrier against environmental aggressors. Therefore, it is crucial that we give it the attention and care it deserves. One way to achieve this is by incorporating natural skincare products into our daily routine.

Natural skincare products are derived from plant-based ingredients and are free from harmful chemicals, synthetic fragrances, and dyes. They are formulated to work in harmony with our skin, providing numerous benefits for all skin types and ages.

First and foremost, natural skincare products are gentle on the skin. Unlike their chemical-laden counterparts, they are less likely to cause irritation, redness, or allergic reactions. This makes them suitable for even the most sensitive skin, including those with conditions such as eczema or rosacea.

Furthermore, natural skincare products are rich in vitamins, minerals, and antioxidants that nourish and rejuvenate the skin. These ingredients help to repair damaged skin cells, reduce the appearance of fine lines and wrinkles, and promote a youthful and radiant complexion. Natural products also contain essential fatty acids, which help to maintain skin elasticity and hydration.

Another significant benefit of natural skincare products is their eco-friendliness. By choosing natural products, we contribute to reducing the amount of harmful chemicals released into the environment during their production and disposal. This helps to preserve the planet's ecosystems and protect its biodiversity for future generations.

Moreover, natural skincare products often have a pleasant and subtle scent derived from essential oils. These natural fragrances not only provide aromatherapy benefits but also eliminate the need for synthetic fragrances, which can irritate the skin and cause allergic reactions.

Lastly, supporting the use of natural skincare products also means supporting sustainable and ethical practices. Many natural skincare brands prioritize fair trade, cruelty-free, and organic ingredients, ensuring that the production process is environmentally responsible and respects the welfare of animals and local communities.

In summary, natural skincare products offer a multitude of benefits for our skin, our health, and the environment. By incorporating them into our skincare routine, we can achieve healthier, more radiant skin while promoting sustainable and ethical practices. So, why not join the green beauty revolution and unleash the power of natural skincare for a better and more beautiful world?

Understanding the Green Beauty Revolution

In recent years, there has been a significant shift in the beauty industry towards natural and sustainable skincare products. This movement, known as the Green Beauty Revolution, has gained momentum and captured the attention of individuals seeking healthier and more environmentally friendly alternatives to traditional skincare.

The Green Beauty Revolution is not just a passing trend; it represents a fundamental shift in the way we perceive and approach skincare. More and more people are becoming aware of the potential harm that synthetic ingredients and harsh chemicals can cause to their skin and overall health. As a result, they are actively seeking out products that are made with natural and organic ingredients.

The term "green beauty" refers to skincare products that are formulated with plant-based ingredients, free from harmful chemicals, and produced in an environmentally conscious manner. These products are not only safer for your skin but also have a lower impact on the planet. By choosing green beauty products, you can take care of your skin while also contributing to a more sustainable future.

One of the main advantages of green beauty is its focus on nourishing and healing the skin. Natural ingredients, such as botanical extracts, essential oils, and antioxidants, are rich in vitamins and minerals that provide numerous benefits to the skin. These ingredients can help hydrate, soothe, and rejuvenate the skin, promoting a healthy and youthful complexion.

Furthermore, green beauty is often cruelty-free, meaning that no animals were harmed during the development and testing of these products. This is an important consideration for individuals who are passionate about animal welfare and want to support brands that align with their values.

Embracing the Green Beauty Revolution is not only beneficial for your skin and the environment but also for your overall well-being. Using natural skincare products can enhance your self-care routine, allowing you to nourish your skin and enjoy a moment of tranquility in your daily life.

Whether you have sensitive skin, acne-prone skin, or are simply looking for a more sustainable skincare alternative, the Green Beauty Revolution has something to offer everyone. By understanding the power of natural skincare and making the switch to green beauty, you can embark on a journey towards healthier and more radiant skin.

In the following chapters, we will delve deeper into the world of green beauty, exploring different natural ingredients, sustainable skincare practices, and the best ways to incorporate green beauty into your daily routine. Get ready to unlock the secrets of the Green Beauty Revolution and unleash the power of natural skincare for a healthier and more beautiful you.

Chapter 2: The Science Behind Natural Skincare

The Harmful Effects of Chemicals in Skincare Products

In today's modern world, where everyone is constantly seeking ways to enhance their beauty and maintain a flawless complexion, it is important to be aware of the potential harmful effects of chemicals found in skincare products. Our skin, being the largest organ of our body, is highly susceptible to absorbing these chemicals, which can have detrimental effects on our overall health and well-being.

Chemicals such as parabens, sulfates, and phthalates, commonly found in many skincare products, have been linked to various health issues. Parabens, for instance, are widely used as preservatives to extend the shelf life of products. However, studies have shown that parabens can disrupt our hormonal balance and potentially lead to reproductive problems and even certain types of cancer. It is alarming to think that the very products we use to enhance our beauty could be causing harm to our bodies.

Sulfates, on the other hand, are responsible for the foaming action in most cleansers and shampoos. While they may give us a satisfying lather, sulfates have been known to strip our skin of its natural oils, leaving it dry, irritated, and prone to inflammation. Additionally, sulfates can penetrate the skin and accumulate in our organs, causing long-term damage.

Phthalates, commonly used in fragrances, have been linked to endocrine disruption, which can lead to hormonal imbalances and reproductive issues. These chemicals are often hidden under the umbrella term "fragrance" on ingredient labels, making it difficult for consumers to make informed choices about the products they use.

Fortunately, there is a growing movement towards green beauty, where natural and organic skincare products are gaining popularity. By opting for these products, we can steer clear of harmful chemicals and embrace the power of natural ingredients that have been used for centuries in traditional skincare practices.

Natural skincare products harness the potent properties of plant extracts, essential oils, and other natural ingredients to nourish and rejuvenate our skin. They promote a holistic approach to beauty, ensuring that our skin is not only healthy on the surface but also from within.

In conclusion, it is crucial for everyone, regardless of their skin type or concerns, to be aware of the harmful effects of chemicals in skincare products. By choosing natural and organic alternatives, we can protect our skin, our health, and contribute to a greener and more sustainable beauty industry. Let us embrace the green beauty revolution and unleash the power of natural skincare for a healthier, more radiant future.

Exploring the Power of Natural Ingredients

In today's fast-paced world, where chemicals and artificial additives seem to dominate every aspect of our lives, it is crucial to take a step back and consider the impact these substances may have on our skin. The beauty industry is no exception, with a plethora of products promising to make us look younger, fresher, and more radiant. However, amidst this sea of synthetic solutions, we often overlook the incredible power and benefits of natural ingredients.

"The Green Beauty Revolution: Unleashing the Power of Natural Skincare" aims to shed light on the magic of Mother Nature and her ability to provide us with all we need to keep our skin healthy, glowing, and vibrant. This subchapter, "Exploring the Power of Natural Ingredients," is a call to embrace the wonders of natural skincare and unlock the potential of our skin.

Natural ingredients are not a new concept; they have been utilized for centuries in various cultures around the world. From traditional herbal remedies to ancient beauty rituals, these ingredients have stood the test of time. They offer a multitude of benefits, such as nourishing and repairing damaged skin, soothing inflammation, and promoting overall skin health.

One of the key advantages of natural ingredients is their ability to work in harmony with our skin, as they are often derived from plants and other organic sources. Unlike their synthetic counterparts, which may cause irritation or disrupt the skin's natural balance, natural ingredients are gentle yet effective. They contain vitamins, minerals, and antioxidants that can help combat signs of aging, reduce acne, and even out skin tone.

This subchapter delves into the world of natural ingredients, showcasing a wide range of options that cater to different skin concerns. From botanical extracts like rosehip oil and aloe vera to nourishing oils such as jojoba and argan, readers will discover the power of these ingredients and how they can transform their skincare routine. Furthermore, it explores the importance of understanding ingredient labels, enabling readers to make informed choices and avoid harmful substances.

"The Green Beauty Revolution" is not just a book for skincare enthusiasts; it is a guide for everyone who wishes to prioritize their skin's health and embrace the beauty nature has to offer. By exploring the power of natural ingredients, readers can embark on a journey towards healthier, more radiant skin, while also contributing to a sustainable and eco-friendly beauty industry.

How Natural Skincare Works with Your Skin

In today's world, where toxins and chemicals seem to be lurking around every corner, it is no wonder that people are becoming more conscious about what they put on their skin. Natural skincare has gained incredible popularity in recent years, and for good reason. It offers a safer and healthier alternative to traditional skincare products, working harmoniously with your skin to enhance its natural beauty.

The human skin is a remarkable organ, capable of healing, protecting, and rejuvenating itself. However, it is also vulnerable to the harmful effects of environmental factors such as pollution and the products we use on a daily basis. Natural skincare works with your skin's inherent abilities to provide it with the nourishment and support it needs to thrive.

One of the key benefits of natural skincare is that it is formulated using ingredients derived from nature, such as plant extracts, essential oils, and botanicals. These ingredients are rich in vitamins, minerals, antioxidants, and other bioactive compounds that have a positive impact on your skin. They work synergistically to address specific skin concerns, such as dryness, acne, or aging, without causing any harm or irritation.

Unlike conventional skincare products that often contain harsh chemicals, synthetic fragrances, and preservatives, natural skincare is free from harmful ingredients. This means that you can use these products with confidence, knowing that they are gentle and safe for your skin. By avoiding toxic chemicals, you are reducing the risk of allergic reactions, sensitivities, and long-term damage to your skin.

Moreover, natural skincare products are designed to support your skin's natural functions. They work to nourish and hydrate your skin, balance its pH levels, and strengthen its protective barrier. By doing so, they help to improve your skin's overall health and vitality, giving you a youthful and radiant complexion.

Another important aspect of natural skincare is its commitment to sustainability and eco-friendliness. Many natural skincare brands prioritize using organic and ethically sourced ingredients, as well as eco-friendly packaging. By choosing natural skincare, you are not only taking care of your skin but also contributing to a healthier planet.

In conclusion, natural skincare is a powerful revolution that is transforming the beauty industry. By understanding how natural skincare works with your skin, you can make informed choices and embrace a safer and more sustainable approach to skincare. Whether you have sensitive, dry, oily, or aging skin, natural skincare has something to offer everyone. So why not join the green beauty revolution and unleash the power of natural skincare for a healthier and more radiant you?

Chapter 3: Building Your Natural Skincare Routine

Assessing Your Skin Type and Concerns

Understanding your skin type and concerns is the first step towards achieving a radiant and healthy complexion. In this subchapter, we will explore the various skin types and common concerns, providing you with the knowledge needed to tailor your skincare routine accordingly.

Every individual has a unique skin type, which can be broadly classified into five categories: oily, dry, combination, sensitive, and normal. Determining your skin type is essential as it enables you to select products that will effectively meet your skin's specific needs.

If you have oily skin, you may notice excess shine, enlarged pores, and a tendency for blemishes. On the other hand, dry skin may feel tight, flaky, and may even experience redness. Combination skin is characterized by an oily T-zone (forehead, nose, and chin) while being normal or dry on the rest of the face. Sensitive skin tends to react easily to various products or environmental factors, often leading to redness, itching, or irritation. Lastly, normal skin is well-balanced, neither too oily nor too dry, with a smooth texture and minimal concerns.

Identifying your skin concerns is equally important. Common concerns include acne, aging, hyperpigmentation, sensitivity, and dehydration. By recognizing these concerns, you can choose targeted products that address the specific issues you wish to tackle.

To assess your skin type and concerns, start by observing your skin's behavior throughout the day. Pay attention to how it feels after cleansing, whether it becomes oily or dry, and if any specific areas are more sensitive than others. Additionally, consider any skin conditions you may be experiencing, such as acne breakouts or signs of aging.

It can also be beneficial to consult with a skincare professional or dermatologist who can perform a thorough analysis of your skin. They will be able to provide expert advice on your skin type, concerns, and recommend suitable skincare products.

Remember, everyone's skin is unique, and it may change over time due to various factors such as age, hormones, or environmental influences. Regularly reassessing your skin type and concerns will ensure that you adjust your skincare routine accordingly, allowing you to achieve and maintain healthy, glowing skin.

In the following chapters, we will delve deeper into each skin type and concern, providing you with tailored advice and product recommendations to address your specific needs. So, get ready to unleash the power of natural skincare and embark on your journey towards a greener and healthier beauty revolution.

Cleansing: The Foundation of Natural Skincare

In our fast-paced world, taking care of our skin is often overlooked. However, the key to achieving healthy and radiant skin lies in a simple yet crucial step: cleansing. Cleansing is the foundation of any skincare routine and plays a vital role in maintaining the health and vitality of our skin. In this subchapter, we will explore the importance of cleansing and how it forms the basis of a natural skincare regimen.

Our skin is constantly exposed to environmental pollutants, dirt, and impurities. These external factors can clog our pores, leading to acne, dullness, and premature aging. Regular cleansing removes these impurities, allowing our skin to breathe and regenerate. Natural skincare advocates for using gentle and plant-based cleansers that effectively remove dirt without stripping the skin of its natural oils.

One of the main benefits of natural cleansers is that they are free from harsh chemicals and synthetic ingredients commonly found in commercial skincare products. Many commercial cleansers contain sulfates, parabens, and artificial fragrances that can irritate the skin and cause long-term damage. Natural cleansers, on the other hand, harness the power of botanical extracts, essential oils, and other natural ingredients to cleanse and nourish the skin without any harmful side effects.

When choosing a cleanser, it is essential to consider your skin type. Those with oily or acne-prone skin may benefit from cleansers containing tea tree oil or witch hazel, known for their antibacterial properties. Dry or sensitive skin, on the other hand, may benefit from gentle cleansers infused with chamomile or aloe vera to soothe and hydrate.

Moreover, cleansing goes beyond just removing surface impurities. It also prepares the skin to absorb the active ingredients in serums, moisturizers, and other skincare products. By cleansing properly, you create a clean canvas for these products to penetrate deep into the skin, maximizing their effectiveness.

In conclusion, cleansing is the cornerstone of any natural skincare routine. By choosing gentle and natural cleansers tailored to your skin type, you can effectively remove impurities, maintain a healthy pH balance, and pave the way for optimal skincare results. Embracing natural skincare practices not only benefits your skin but also contributes to a healthier and more sustainable planet. So, start your skincare revolution today by embracing the power of cleansing and unlock the natural beauty within you.

Nourishing Your Skin with Natural Moisturizers

In today's fast-paced world, it's no secret that our skin often bears the brunt of our busy lives. With pollution, stress, and harsh weather conditions, it's no wonder our skin can become dull, dry, and lackluster. However, there is a simple and effective solution to restore your skin's natural radiance – natural moisturizers.

In this subchapter, we will explore the power of natural moisturizers and how they can transform your skin. Whether you have dry, oily, or combination skin, these nourishing ingredients will work wonders for you.

One of the key benefits of natural moisturizers is their ability to hydrate the skin deeply. Unlike synthetic products that may contain harmful chemicals, natural moisturizers are packed with vitamins, antioxidants, and essential fatty acids that penetrate the skin's layers, providing intense hydration and nourishment. This helps to improve the skin's elasticity, reduce the appearance of fine lines and wrinkles, and leave your skin looking plump and youthful.

Another advantage of natural moisturizers is their ability to soothe and calm irritated skin. Many plant-based ingredients, such as aloe vera, chamomile, and lavender, possess anti-inflammatory properties that can help reduce redness, irritation, and acne. By opting for natural moisturizers, you can say goodbye to harsh chemicals that may further aggravate your skin condition.

Furthermore, natural moisturizers often contain natural oils that mimic the skin's natural sebum. This means they can help regulate oil production, balance the skin's pH levels, and prevent clogged pores. If you struggle with oily or acne-prone skin, incorporating natural moisturizers into your skincare routine can help restore harmony and promote a clearer complexion.

When selecting natural moisturizers, it's essential to consider your skin type and specific concerns. Look for ingredients like shea butter, jojoba oil, coconut oil, and hyaluronic acid, which are known for their moisturizing properties. Additionally, opt for organic and sustainably sourced products to ensure you're not only caring for your skin but also the environment.

In conclusion, nourishing your skin with natural moisturizers is a vital step in your skincare routine. By harnessing the power of nature's ingredients, you can achieve a healthy, radiant complexion while avoiding harmful chemicals. So, why wait? Embrace the green beauty revolution and unlock the transformative potential of natural skincare today. Your skin will thank you!

Targeted Treatments for Common Skin Issues

When it comes to taking care of our skin, we all want effective and natural solutions that will address our specific concerns. Thankfully, the world of green beauty offers a range of targeted treatments for common skin issues, providing a holistic approach to skincare that can benefit everyone.

Acne is a prevalent skin problem that affects people of all ages. Traditional treatments often contain harsh chemicals that can strip the skin of its natural oils, leading to dryness and irritation. However, the green beauty revolution has introduced natural alternatives that are just as effective, if not more so. Ingredients like tea tree oil, witch hazel, and aloe vera have proven anti-inflammatory and antibacterial properties, making them excellent choices for treating acne. These ingredients can unclog pores, reduce redness, and promote healing without harming the skin's natural balance.

Another common concern is dry skin, which can often lead to roughness, flakiness, and discomfort. Many conventional moisturizers contain synthetic ingredients that can create a temporary illusion of hydration but fail to nourish the skin in the long run. Natural alternatives such as shea butter, coconut oil, and jojoba oil are rich in essential fatty acids and vitamins that deeply hydrate the skin, restoring its natural moisture barrier. These ingredients penetrate the skin's layers, providing long-lasting hydration and leaving it soft and supple.

Sensitive skin requires extra care and attention. Harsh chemicals and fragrances found in many skincare products can cause irritation and redness. The green beauty approach focuses on gentle and soothing ingredients like chamomile, oatmeal, and lavender, which calm and nourish sensitive skin. These ingredients have anti-inflammatory properties that help reduce redness and promote skin healing, making them ideal choices for those with sensitive skin.

Addressing specific skin concerns like hyperpigmentation, wrinkles, and sun damage is also possible with targeted treatments from the green beauty world. Natural ingredients like rosehip oil, vitamin C, and licorice root extract have been proven to fade dark spots, boost collagen production, and protect the skin from the harmful effects of UV rays. These ingredients provide a natural and effective solution for achieving a more even complexion and reducing the signs of aging.

By harnessing the power of natural ingredients, targeted treatments for common skin issues offer a more sustainable and safer approach to skincare. Embracing the green beauty revolution allows us to nourish and care for our skin while avoiding harmful chemicals and promoting overall skin health. Whether you're struggling with acne, dryness, sensitivity, or specific concerns, there is a green beauty solution out there that can unlock the potential for radiant and healthy skin.

Chapter 4: DIY Natural Skincare Recipes

The Benefits of Making Your Own Skincare Products

In today's world, where the beauty industry bombards us with countless skincare products containing harmful chemicals and artificial ingredients, it is essential to explore alternative options that prioritize our skin's health. One such option is making your own skincare products using natural ingredients. By doing so, you not only take control of what goes into your skincare routine but also reap numerous benefits for your skin. Let's delve into the advantages of embracing this green beauty revolution.

First and foremost, making your own skincare products allows you to avoid harmful chemicals commonly found in commercial products. Many store-bought skincare items contain parabens, sulfates, and artificial fragrances that can irritate and damage your skin over time. By using natural ingredients such as essential oils, plant extracts, and organic butters, you can create products that nourish, protect, and rejuvenate your skin without any harmful side effects.

Additionally, creating your skincare products gives you the flexibility to tailor them to your specific skin type and concerns. Whether you have dry, sensitive, oily, or acne-prone skin, the ability to customize your skincare regimen ensures that you address your unique needs effectively. You can experiment with different combinations of ingredients until you find the perfect formula that works for you, helping to achieve healthier and more radiant skin.

Moreover, making your own skincare products is not only beneficial for your skin but also for the environment. Commercial skincare production often contributes to pollution, excessive packaging, and unethical practices. By opting for homemade products, you reduce your carbon footprint and minimize waste. You can reuse and recycle containers, choose sustainable ingredients, and support local suppliers, creating a positive impact on both your skin and the planet.

Furthermore, making your own skincare products can be a fun and rewarding experience. It allows you to tap into your creativity, explore natural remedies, and indulge in self-care practices. Mixing your unique blends of ingredients, experimenting with different scents and textures, and pampering yourself with homemade treatments can be a therapeutic and empowering process. It gives you a sense of ownership over your skincare routine, elevating it from a mundane task to a delightful ritual.

In conclusion, making your own skincare products offers numerous benefits for your skin, your health, and the environment. From avoiding harmful chemicals to tailoring products to suit your skin type, embracing the green beauty revolution empowers you to take charge of your skincare journey. So why not embark on this natural skincare adventure and unlock the power of green beauty? Your skin will thank you.

Essential Oils for Skincare

In the quest for healthier, more radiant skin, many people are turning to natural remedies that can nourish and rejuvenate their skin without the use of harsh chemicals. Essential oils have gained popularity in recent years for their numerous skincare benefits. These potent extracts from plants not only smell amazing but also possess remarkable properties that can help address various skin concerns.

One of the most significant advantages of using essential oils for skincare is their ability to moisturize and hydrate the skin. Many essential oils, such as lavender, chamomile, and rose, have powerful moisturizing properties that can help combat dryness and maintain the skin's natural moisture balance. These oils can be particularly beneficial for individuals with dry or dehydrated skin, as they provide deep hydration and promote a soft, supple complexion.

Another remarkable benefit of essential oils is their ability to soothe and calm irritated skin. Tea tree oil, for example, is well-known for its anti-inflammatory and antimicrobial properties, making it an excellent choice for individuals with acne-prone or sensitive skin. Similarly, chamomile and rosemary essential oils can help reduce redness and inflammation, providing relief for those with rosacea or other skin conditions.

Essential oils also possess potent antioxidant properties, which can help protect the skin from environmental damage and premature aging. Oils such as frankincense, geranium, and neroli are rich in antioxidants that neutralize free radicals and promote a youthful complexion. These oils can help minimize the appearance of fine lines, wrinkles, and age spots, giving your skin a radiant, more youthful appearance.

When using essential oils for skincare, it's important to dilute them properly before applying them to the skin. Essential oils are highly concentrated, and direct application can cause skin irritation. Diluting them with carrier oils like jojoba, almond, or coconut oil ensures safe and effective use.

Incorporating essential oils into your skincare routine can be a game-changer, offering natural and effective solutions for various skin concerns. However, it's crucial to remember that everyone's skin is unique, and what works for one person may not work for another. It's recommended to conduct a patch test before using any new essential oil to check for allergies or sensitivities.

In conclusion, essential oils offer a natural and holistic approach to skincare. From moisturizing and hydrating to soothing and protecting, these potent extracts have the potential to transform your skincare routine. Embrace the power of essential oils and unlock the secret to healthier, more radiant skin.

Homemade Facial Cleansers and Exfoliators

When it comes to achieving healthy and radiant skin, commercial skincare products often fall short of expectations. Many contain harsh chemicals and artificial ingredients that can do more harm than good. Fortunately, there is a natural and affordable alternative – homemade facial cleansers and exfoliators. In this subchapter, we will explore the power of these DIY skincare solutions and how they can transform your skin.

Facial cleansers are an essential part of any skincare routine. They help remove dirt, grime, and makeup, leaving your skin clean and refreshed. But why settle for store-bought cleansers when you can easily make your own at home? Using simple and natural ingredients, such as honey, coconut oil, or aloe vera, you can create personalized cleansers that cater to your unique skin type. Whether you have dry, oily, or sensitive skin, there is a homemade cleanser for everyone.

Exfoliating is another crucial step in maintaining healthy skin. Regular exfoliation helps remove dead skin cells, unclog pores, and promote smoother, more radiant skin. Instead of relying on abrasive scrubs that can damage your skin, why not try making your own gentle and effective exfoliators? With ingredients like sugar, coffee grounds, or oatmeal, you can create exfoliators that not only buff away dead skin but also nourish and rejuvenate your complexion.

The benefits of homemade facial cleansers and exfoliators extend beyond their natural and gentle formulas. By making your own skincare products, you have full control over the ingredients you use, ensuring that no harmful chemicals touch your skin. Additionally, homemade solutions are often more cost-effective than their commercial counterparts, saving you money in the long run.

In this subchapter, we will provide easy-to-follow recipes and step-by-step instructions for creating a variety of homemade facial cleansers and exfoliators. We will also discuss the specific benefits of each ingredient, allowing you to choose the ones that best suit your skin's needs. Whether you are seeking a deep-cleansing charcoal scrub, a soothing oatmeal cleanser, or a brightening citrus exfoliator, you will find a wealth of options to explore.

Embrace the power of natural skincare and discover the transformative effects of homemade facial cleansers and exfoliators. Unlock the secrets to healthy and glowing skin with ingredients straight from your pantry or garden. Join the green beauty revolution and take control of your skincare routine today.

DIY Face Masks and Serums

In this subchapter, we will delve into the exciting world of DIY face masks and serums, empowering you to unlock the potential of natural skincare. Whether you are a skincare enthusiast or someone who simply wants to pamper their skin, this section has something for everyone.

Face masks are a fantastic way to rejuvenate and nourish your skin. They can address specific concerns such as acne, dryness, or dullness. By using natural ingredients readily available in your kitchen, you can create personalized masks tailored to your skin's unique needs.

For those struggling with acne, a DIY face mask with honey, tea tree oil, and aloe vera can work wonders. Honey has antibacterial properties, while tea tree oil and aloe vera soothe inflammation and promote healing. Mixing these ingredients together creates a potent mask that can reduce redness and blemishes.

If your skin tends to be dry, a face mask with avocado, yogurt, and honey can provide intense hydration. Avocado is rich in healthy fats that nourish and moisturize the skin, while yogurt and honey soothe and soften. This mask will leave your skin feeling plump, smooth, and revitalized.

Serums, on the other hand, are lightweight formulations that penetrate deep into the skin, delivering concentrated nutrients. They can target specific skin issues such as wrinkles, hyperpigmentation, or uneven texture. Creating your own serums allows you to tailor the ingredients to your skin's unique requirements.

For example, a DIY serum with rosehip oil, vitamin E, and lavender oil can combat signs of aging. Rosehip oil is packed with antioxidants that promote collagen production, while vitamin E and lavender oil soothe and protect the skin. This serum can help reduce the appearance of wrinkles and improve overall skin texture.

Remember, before applying any homemade face masks or serums, it is crucial to perform a patch test to check for any allergies or sensitivities. Additionally, always use fresh and high-quality ingredients to ensure optimal results.

By exploring the world of DIY face masks and serums, you can incorporate natural skincare into your daily routine, giving your skin the love and care it deserves. So, unleash your creativity, experiment with different ingredients, and discover the power of Green Beauty Revolution for yourself! Your skin will thank you!

Chapter 5: Shopping for Natural Skincare Products

Understanding Labels: Decoding Green Beauty Jargon

In this subchapter, we will delve into the complex world of green beauty and decipher the jargon commonly found on skincare product labels. With the increasing popularity of natural skincare, it is crucial for everyone, especially those with specific skin concerns, to understand the ingredients and claims made by brands. By decoding the green beauty jargon, you can make informed decisions and embrace the power of natural skincare.

1. Ingredients to Look for:

a. Organic: This term refers to ingredients that have been grown without the use of synthetic fertilizers, pesticides, or genetically modified organisms (GMOs). Look for certifications such as USDA Organic or Ecocert to ensure authenticity.

b. Natural: Products labeled as natural should ideally contain ingredients derived from nature, such as plant extracts, essential oils, and minerals. However, be cautious as this term is not regulated and can sometimes be misleading.

c. Cruelty-Free: This label indicates that no animals were harmed during the production or testing of the product. Look for certifications like Leaping Bunny or PETA's Cruelty-Free logo.

2. Common Claims:

a. Paraben-Free: Parabens are synthetic preservatives that have been linked to hormonal disruption. Choosing paraben-free products can minimize potential risks.

b. Sulfate-Free: Sulfates are harsh detergents commonly found in cleansers and shampoos. They can strip the skin of its natural oils, leading to dryness and irritation. Opting for sulfate-free products can be gentler on the skin.

c. Vegan: Vegan products do not contain any animal-derived ingredients or by-products. They are suitable for those following a vegan lifestyle or individuals with specific allergies and sensitivities.

3. Greenwashing:

Greenwashing refers to misleading marketing tactics used by some brands to make their products appear more environmentally friendly or natural than they actually are. To identify greenwashing, look for certifications from reputable organizations, read ingredient lists carefully, and research the brand's sustainability practices.

Understanding labels and decoding green beauty jargon is essential for anyone interested in prioritizing natural skincare. By being aware of the ingredients and claims made by brands, you can make conscious choices that align with your skin's needs and ethical values. Remember, knowledge is power, and with the right information, you can embark on a green beauty revolution that benefits both your skin and the environment.

Choosing the Right Brands and Ingredients

In today's world, where the demand for natural and sustainable products is on the rise, it is crucial to make informed choices when it comes to skincare. With a plethora of brands and ingredients available, it can be overwhelming to navigate through the options. However, understanding how to choose the right brands and ingredients can make all the difference in achieving healthy, radiant skin.

When it comes to selecting brands, it is essential to prioritize those that promote transparency and sustainability. Look for brands that are committed to using natural, organic, and ethically sourced ingredients. These brands often have certifications or labels that guarantee their products are free from harmful chemicals and have been produced with minimal impact on the environment.

Researching the brand's values and mission can provide insight into their commitment to green beauty. Check if they are cruelty-free, meaning they do not test on animals, and if they use environmentally friendly packaging. Remember, supporting brands that align with your values not only benefits your skin but also contributes to a more sustainable future.

Equally important is understanding the ingredients used in skincare products. Avoid products that contain harsh chemicals, synthetic fragrances, and parabens, as these can be harmful to your skin and overall health. Instead, opt for products with plant-based ingredients, such as aloe vera, chamomile, and green tea, which have nourishing and soothing properties.

Reading product labels is crucial in deciphering the ingredients used. Be cautious of greenwashing, a marketing tactic where brands use misleading claims to appear more environmentally friendly. Look for specific certifications like USDA Organic, Ecocert, or COSMOS to ensure the product meets rigorous standards.

Consider your skin type and concerns when choosing ingredients. For example, if you have dry skin, look for ingredients like hyaluronic acid and shea butter to provide intense hydration. If you struggle with acne-prone skin, ingredients like tea tree oil and salicylic acid can help combat breakouts.

Ultimately, choosing the right brands and ingredients requires research and experimentation. Don't be afraid to try different products and see how your skin responds. Remember, the journey to green beauty is a personal one, and finding what works best for you will result in healthier, happier skin.

By taking the time to choose brands committed to sustainability and understanding the power of natural ingredients, you can revolutionize your skincare routine. Embrace the green beauty revolution and unleash the potential of natural skincare for a more radiant and healthier you.

Where to Buy Natural Skincare Products

In today's world, where harmful chemicals and synthetic ingredients have become all too common in skincare products, more and more people are turning to natural alternatives. If you're concerned about the health and appearance of your skin, it's important to know where you can find high-quality, natural skincare products. In this subchapter, we will explore various avenues for purchasing these products, ensuring that you can make informed decisions and embrace the green beauty revolution.

1. Specialty Stores: One of the most accessible places to find natural skincare products is your local health food or wellness store. These stores typically have dedicated sections for natural beauty products, showcasing a wide range of brands that prioritize organic and plant-based ingredients. The advantage of shopping in-store is that you can physically examine and test the products before making a purchase.

2. Online Retailers: The internet has opened up a vast world of options for purchasing natural skincare products. Online retailers like Amazon, Sephora, and Ulta Beauty offer a diverse selection of brands and products, often accompanied by customer reviews that can help you make an informed choice. Keep in mind that it's essential to read the ingredient lists and research the brands to ensure they align with your values.

3. Brand Websites: Many natural skincare brands have their own websites, where you can directly purchase their products. This allows you to learn more about the brand's philosophy, ingredient sourcing, and manufacturing processes. Additionally, some brands offer

exclusive discounts, bundle deals, or loyalty programs on their websites, making it a cost-effective option.

4. Farmers' Markets and Local Artisanal Shops: If you prefer to support local businesses and enjoy a more personalized shopping experience, farmers' markets and local artisanal shops are excellent options. These venues often feature small-scale skincare brands that prioritize sustainability and use locally sourced ingredients. Interacting with the brand owners or representatives can provide valuable insights into their product formulation and ethos.

5. Subscription Boxes: For those who love surprises and discovering new products, subscription boxes dedicated to natural skincare can be a great option. These curated boxes often contain a selection of full-sized or sample-sized products from various brands, allowing you to try them out before committing to a full-size purchase.

Remember, when purchasing natural skincare products, always prioritize brands that are transparent about their ingredients, manufacturing processes, and sustainability efforts. By making informed choices and embracing the green beauty revolution, you can nourish your skin while contributing to a healthier planet.

Evaluating Product Claims and Certifications

In today's world, where the beauty industry is flooded with countless skincare products, it's becoming increasingly important to be able to distinguish between genuine claims and clever marketing tactics. As consumers, we are bombarded with promises of youthful, radiant skin, but how do we know which products truly deliver on their claims? This subchapter aims to equip you with the knowledge and tools necessary to evaluate product claims and certifications, ensuring that you make informed choices for your skin.

When evaluating product claims, it's crucial to do your research and not blindly trust everything you read. Look beyond catchy slogans and flashy packaging, and instead focus on the ingredients list. Understanding the ingredients can provide valuable insights into the effectiveness and potential side effects of a product. Educate yourself about commonly used ingredients, such as antioxidants, hyaluronic acid, and plant extracts, to determine their benefits for your specific skin concerns.

Furthermore, certifications play a vital role in verifying a product's authenticity and credibility. Look for recognized certifications like USDA Organic, COSMOS, or Leaping Bunny, as they ensure that the product meets certain standards of quality, safety, and sustainability. These certifications indicate that the brand has undergone rigorous testing and adheres to strict guidelines, giving you peace of mind that you're making a conscious choice for both your skin and the environment.

However, it's important to note that not all certifications are created equal. Some brands may employ their own in-house certifications that lack independent verification. Be cautious of such certifications and do your due diligence by researching the certifying body's credibility and transparency.

To further evaluate a product, consider checking online reviews from trusted sources or seeking recommendations from skincare experts. Real-life experiences and feedback from other users can help you gauge the effectiveness of a product and its compatibility with different skin types.

Remember, as a consumer, you hold the power to make informed decisions and demand transparency from skincare brands. By evaluating product claims and certifications, you can navigate the overwhelming beauty market and choose products that truly deliver on their promises, while prioritizing the health and well-being of your skin.

In conclusion, understanding how to evaluate product claims and certifications is essential in the pursuit of a green beauty revolution. By being mindful of ingredients, seeking reputable certifications, and considering real-life experiences, you can confidently choose skincare products that align with your skin's needs and contribute to a healthier, more sustainable future. Empower yourself with knowledge and take control of your skincare journey.

Chapter 6: Overcoming Challenges in the Green Beauty Journey

Dealing with Transitioning Periods

Transitioning periods are inevitable in life, and when it comes to our skin, they can often be quite challenging. Whether it's due to seasonal changes, hormonal fluctuations, or lifestyle adjustments, our skin can react in unexpected ways. However, understanding and effectively managing these transitions can help maintain a healthy and radiant complexion. In this subchapter, we will explore various strategies for dealing with transitioning periods and provide practical tips to address common skin concerns.

First and foremost, it's essential to listen to your skin. Pay attention to any changes, such as increased dryness, breakouts, or sensitivity. By understanding the root cause behind these issues, you can tailor your skincare routine accordingly. For instance, during colder months, your skin may require richer and more nourishing products to combat dryness. Similarly, if you're experiencing hormonal changes, incorporating calming ingredients like chamomile or lavender can help soothe inflammation.

Another crucial aspect of managing transitioning periods is maintaining a consistent skincare routine. It's tempting to experiment with various products or abandon your routine altogether when faced with skin challenges. However, this can further disrupt your skin's equilibrium. Stick to a gentle cleanser, moisturizer, and sunscreen as the foundation of your routine, and gradually introduce new products or treatments to avoid overwhelming your skin.

Additionally, adjusting your diet and lifestyle can greatly impact your skin's health during transitioning periods. Proper hydration, a balanced diet rich in antioxidants, and regular exercise can enhance your skin's natural radiance. Incorporating stress management techniques like meditation or yoga can also help reduce the impact of emotional and environmental stressors on your skin.

When dealing with transitioning periods, it's crucial to be patient and give your skin time to adjust. Results may not be immediate, and it's important not to lose hope. Remember, every individual's skin is unique, and what works for someone else may not work for you. Be open to experimenting with different natural skincare products, but always prioritize those that are gentle and free from harmful chemicals.

By following these tips and embracing the power of natural skincare, you can navigate through transitioning periods with confidence and grace. Remember, your skin is a reflection of your overall well-being, so take the time to care for it and embrace the beauty revolution that comes with it.

Addressing the Myth of Natural Skincare Inefficiency

In recent years, the popularity of natural skincare products has skyrocketed, with more and more individuals opting for a healthier and more sustainable approach to their skincare routines. However, there still persists a myth that natural skincare is less effective than its chemical-laden counterparts. This subchapter aims to debunk this misconception and shed light on the true power of natural skincare.

One of the main factors contributing to the belief in the inefficiency of natural skincare is the misconception that only synthetic ingredients can deliver visible results. This couldn't be further from the truth. Natural skincare products harness the power of botanical extracts, organic oils, and plant-based ingredients that have been used for centuries for their healing and rejuvenating properties. These ingredients work in harmony with the skin, providing essential nutrients, antioxidants, and hydration that promote a healthy complexion.

Moreover, natural skincare products are free from harmful chemicals such as parabens, sulfates, and synthetic fragrances that can irritate and damage the skin in the long run. By avoiding these harmful substances, natural skincare allows the skin to breathe and heal, leading to a clearer and more radiant complexion.

Additionally, natural skincare products often undergo rigorous testing and quality control to ensure their effectiveness. Many reputable natural skincare brands invest in scientific research and development, ensuring that their formulas are backed by scientific evidence and clinical trials. This dedication to efficacy and transparency sets natural skincare apart from its chemical-laden counterparts.

It is also important to note that natural skincare is not a one-size-fits-all solution. Just like any other skincare routine, it requires understanding your skin's unique needs and choosing products that specifically target those concerns. Natural skincare offers a wide range of products tailored to different skin types, whether you have oily, dry, sensitive, or combination skin.

In conclusion, the myth of natural skincare inefficiency is just that - a myth. Natural skincare products are not only effective but also provide numerous benefits for your skin and overall well-being. By embracing natural skincare, you can achieve a healthier, more radiant complexion while also contributing to a greener and more sustainable future for our planet. It's time to unleash the power of natural skincare and revolutionize your beauty routine.

Overcoming Price and Accessibility Concerns

In today's fast-paced world, more and more individuals are becoming conscious about the products they use on their skin. The desire to embrace natural skincare has gained considerable momentum, as people are increasingly aware of the potential harm that synthetic ingredients can cause. However, two major concerns often hinder individuals from fully embracing the green beauty revolution – price and accessibility.

Price is a common concern for many when it comes to natural skincare. It is true that some natural and organic products can be more expensive than their conventional counterparts. However, it is essential to understand that investing in your skin's health is a long-term commitment. By prioritizing quality over quantity, you can minimize the potential damage caused by harsh chemicals and toxins found in conventional skincare products. Besides, natural skincare products tend to be more concentrated, meaning you need less product for the same effect. Thus, the initial investment can actually be more cost-effective in the long run.

Fortunately, the green beauty market is expanding rapidly, leading to increased accessibility for all. While it may have been challenging to find natural skincare products in the past, today, there are numerous options available both online and in physical stores. Many brands are dedicated to making natural skincare accessible to everyone, offering a wide range of products at various price points. Additionally, with the rise of social media and online communities, it has become easier than ever to discover and connect with like-minded individuals who can recommend affordable, high-quality natural skincare products.

Moreover, embracing the green beauty revolution doesn't necessarily mean completely abandoning your existing skincare routine. Gradually incorporating natural products into your regimen can be a more budget-friendly approach. Start by replacing one or two products at a time, such as cleansers or moisturizers, with natural alternatives. This allows you to gauge the effectiveness and compatibility of the products with your skin before making a full transition.

Remember, your skin is an investment, and prioritizing its health will pay off in the long run. Overcoming price and accessibility concerns is not only possible but also necessary for the overall well-being of your skin. By making informed choices and gradually incorporating natural skincare products into your routine, you can unleash the power of natural ingredients and embark on a green beauty revolution that is accessible to everyone.

Sustainable Packaging and Eco-Friendly Practices

In today's world, where environmental consciousness is on the rise, it is crucial for industries to adopt sustainable practices that contribute to a greener and healthier planet. The skincare industry is no exception. With the growing awareness of the impact of consumerism on the environment, consumers are demanding sustainable packaging and eco-friendly practices from the brands they trust. In this subchapter, we will explore the significance of sustainable packaging and the role it plays in the green beauty revolution.

When it comes to skincare, packaging serves a vital purpose in preserving the integrity of the products and ensuring their safety and longevity. However, traditional packaging materials like plastic, which take centuries to decompose, have a devastating impact on the environment. This is where sustainable packaging comes into play. It involves using recyclable, biodegradable, and renewable materials that have a reduced carbon footprint.

One of the most popular alternatives to traditional packaging is glass. Glass is not only recyclable but also preserves the quality of the products by protecting them from sunlight and air exposure. It is an excellent option for skincare products as it is non-reactive, ensuring the products remain fresh and potent for longer periods. Additionally, glass packaging can be repurposed or recycled, minimizing waste and reducing the overall environmental impact.

Another sustainable packaging option gaining popularity is using post-consumer recycled (PCR) materials. By incorporating recycled materials into packaging, brands can significantly reduce their carbon footprint. Additionally, choosing materials that are easily recyclable, such as paper or cardboard, can further contribute to eco-friendly practices. These materials can be recycled multiple times, reducing the demand for virgin materials.

Eco-friendly practices extend beyond packaging materials. Brands can also focus on reducing their overall environmental impact through various initiatives. For instance, implementing refillable packaging systems allows customers to reuse containers, significantly reducing waste. Brands can also minimize their carbon footprint by sourcing ingredients locally, reducing transportation emissions.

In conclusion, sustainable packaging and eco-friendly practices are essential components of the green beauty revolution. By adopting these practices, skincare brands can make a positive impact on the environment and align themselves with the growing consumer demand for eco-conscious products. As consumers, it is crucial for us to support brands that prioritize sustainability, as our choices have the power to shape a greener future for our planet. Together, we can unleash the power of natural skincare while preserving the beauty of our environment for generations to come.

Chapter 7: The Future of Natural Skincare

Innovations in Natural Skincare Technology

In recent years, there has been a remarkable shift in the beauty industry towards natural skincare products. People from all walks of life, regardless of age or gender, are becoming increasingly aware of the harmful effects that synthetic chemicals can have on their skin. As a result, the demand for innovative and effective natural skincare solutions is skyrocketing.

The field of natural skincare technology has seen remarkable advancements, offering a plethora of options for those seeking healthier and more sustainable alternatives. From plant-based ingredients to cutting-edge extraction methods, these innovations are revolutionizing the way we care for our skin.

One of the most exciting developments in natural skincare technology is the use of potent botanical extracts. Scientists have discovered that plants possess an astonishing array of beneficial compounds that can nourish, repair, and protect the skin. These extracts, obtained through sustainable and eco-friendly methods, are now being incorporated into a wide range of skincare products. Whether it's aloe vera to soothe inflammation, green tea to combat free radicals, or chamomile to calm sensitive skin, these natural ingredients are proving to be powerful allies in our quest for radiant and healthy skin.

Another notable innovation is the use of advanced extraction techniques. Traditionally, natural skincare products were made by steeping herbs in oil or water. However, modern technology has allowed for the development of more efficient methods that preserve the potency of the plant's active compounds. For example, supercritical CO2 extraction utilizes carbon dioxide in its liquid state to extract the desired components from plants without the need for harmful solvents. This process ensures a higher concentration of beneficial compounds, resulting in more effective skincare products.

Furthermore, advancements in natural preservatives have addressed one of the major concerns associated with natural skincare products. Historically, the limited shelf life of natural ingredients has posed challenges for manufacturers. However, innovative techniques such as airless packaging and the use of natural preservatives derived from plants have extended the shelf life of these products without compromising their integrity. This means that consumers can now enjoy the benefits of natural skincare products for longer periods, without the worry of spoilage or reduced effectiveness.

As the green beauty revolution continues to gain momentum, innovations in natural skincare technology are redefining the way we approach our skincare routines. With a focus on sustainability, efficacy, and safety, these advancements offer a promising future for everyone seeking healthier, more radiant skin. By embracing these innovations, we can unleash the power of natural skincare and embark on a journey towards a more beautiful and sustainable world.

The Role of Science and Research in Green Beauty

In today's world, where the demand for natural and sustainable products is on the rise, it is crucial to understand the role of science and research in the realm of green beauty. When it comes to skincare, science plays a pivotal role in developing effective and safe products that cater to the needs of our skin while minimizing the impact on the environment.

Scientific research allows us to delve deep into the properties of natural ingredients and their potential benefits for our skin. Through rigorous testing and analysis, scientists are able to identify the active compounds present in plants, herbs, and other natural resources. This knowledge enables formulators to create skincare products that harness the power of nature while delivering visible results.

One of the key advantages of science-backed green beauty is the ability to understand the mechanisms behind skincare. Researchers can investigate how certain ingredients interact with our skin cells, ensuring that products are not only gentle but also capable of addressing specific concerns such as acne, aging, or sensitivity. This knowledge empowers individuals to make informed choices about the products they use, ultimately leading to healthier and happier skin.

Moreover, scientific research provides valuable insights into the environmental impact of skincare products. It allows us to assess the sustainability of various manufacturing processes, packaging materials, and ingredient sourcing methods. By understanding the lifecycle of a product, researchers can suggest eco-friendly alternatives, reducing waste and conserving resources.

Science also plays a crucial role in debunking myths and misconceptions surrounding green beauty. It provides evidence-based information to differentiate between marketing gimmicks and genuine claims. Through scientific studies, we can determine the safety and efficacy of certain ingredients, ensuring that we make informed decisions about what we put on our skin.

As consumers, it is important to recognize the significance of supporting brands that invest in scientific research. By doing so, we encourage innovation, transparency, and the development of sustainable and effective green beauty products. We have the power to drive positive change through our choices.

In conclusion, science and research are integral to the green beauty revolution. They allow us to harness the power of nature while ensuring that our skincare products are safe, effective, and sustainable. By embracing science-backed green beauty, we can nurture our skin, protect the environment, and contribute to a healthier and more beautiful world for everyone.

Advocating for Transparency and Regulation in the Industry

In recent years, the skincare industry has witnessed a surge in demand for natural and organic products. Consumers are becoming more conscious about what they put on their skin, seeking out safer and healthier alternatives to traditional skincare products. This shift is not just a passing trend; it represents a growing movement towards clean beauty and the desire for transparency and regulation in the industry.

Transparency is crucial when it comes to skincare products. Consumers have the right to know exactly what ingredients are present in the products they use, and how these ingredients may affect their skin and overall health. Unfortunately, the skincare industry has long been plagued by a lack of transparency, with many products containing harmful chemicals and potentially toxic substances. This is why advocating for transparency in the industry is so vital.

By advocating for transparency, we empower consumers to make informed choices about the products they purchase and use on their skin. When consumers have access to detailed ingredient lists and are aware of the potential risks associated with certain chemicals, they can make decisions that align with their personal values and health goals. This not only promotes healthier skin, but also encourages companies to prioritize the use of safe and natural ingredients.

Regulation is another crucial aspect of the skincare industry. While some companies voluntarily adopt clean and natural practices, others continue to use harmful ingredients without consequence. By advocating for regulation, we can ensure that all skincare products undergo rigorous testing and meet stringent safety standards. This will help eliminate the use of potentially harmful chemicals and protect the well-being of consumers.

Regulation also fosters innovation and encourages the development of safer alternatives. When companies are held accountable for the ingredients they use, they are prompted to invest in research and development to create effective and natural skincare solutions. This benefits both the industry and consumers, as it supports the growth of sustainable and ethical practices.

In conclusion, advocating for transparency and regulation in the skincare industry is essential for the health and well-being of consumers. By demanding transparency, we can make informed choices about the products we use on our skin. Simultaneously, by pushing for regulation, we can ensure that all skincare products meet strict safety standards and foster the growth of the clean beauty movement. Let us come together as individuals, demand transparency, and advocate for a regulated industry that prioritizes the health and beauty of our skin.

Embracing a Holistic Approach to Natural Beauty

In today's fast-paced world, many of us are seeking ways to improve our overall well-being, including the health and appearance of our skin. The Green Beauty Revolution: Unleashing the Power of Natural Skincare offers a comprehensive guide to embracing a holistic approach to natural beauty that will benefit everyone, regardless of age, gender, or skin type.

When it comes to skincare, many of us focus solely on external treatments. We invest in expensive products promising instant results, without considering the underlying factors that contribute to the health and vitality of our skin. However, true beauty goes beyond what meets the eye. It is time to shift our mindset and adopt a holistic approach to skincare.

Holistic skincare emphasizes the connection between our skin, body, and mind. It recognizes that our skin is a reflection of our overall health and well-being. By addressing the root causes of skin issues and nourishing our bodies from within, we can achieve long-lasting and radiant results.

This subchapter delves into the importance of embracing a holistic approach to natural beauty. It explores the interconnectedness of our skin with our diet, lifestyle, and emotional well-being. By understanding the impact of these factors, we can make informed choices regarding our skincare routine and overall lifestyle.

We will explore the power of nutrition and how certain foods can promote healthy skin from the inside out. We will delve into the benefits of incorporating mindful practices such as meditation and stress reduction techniques to promote emotional well-being, which in turn benefits our skin.

Moreover, this subchapter will guide you through the process of creating a personalized skincare routine using natural and eco-friendly products. It will provide tips on how to identify harmful ingredients commonly found in conventional skincare products and offer alternatives that are gentle on your skin and the environment.

Embracing a holistic approach to natural beauty is not a quick fix, but rather a journey towards sustainable self-care. By considering our skin as an integral part of our overall well-being, we can achieve a radiant complexion that reflects our inner vitality and harmony.

Whether you are a skincare enthusiast or a beginner, this subchapter is designed to empower you to take charge of your skin health and embrace a holistic approach to natural beauty. It is time to unlock the power within and embark on a transformative journey towards radiant and sustainable self-care.

Chapter 8: Inspiring Success Stories in Natural Skincare

Entrepreneurs and Brands Leading the Green Beauty Revolution

In recent years, there has been a significant shift in the beauty industry towards more sustainable and eco-friendly practices. Consumers are becoming increasingly aware of the negative impacts that conventional beauty products can have on their skin and the environment. As a result, a new wave of entrepreneurs and brands dedicated to the green beauty movement has emerged, revolutionizing the way we approach skincare.

These entrepreneurs and brands are passionate about creating products that are not only effective but also safe and sustainable. They prioritize using natural and organic ingredients, avoiding harmful chemicals, and minimizing their environmental footprint. Their mission is to provide consumers with skincare options that promote both inner and outer beauty, while also protecting the planet.

One of the leading entrepreneurs in this green beauty revolution is Jane Smith, founder of a renowned skincare brand. Jane's journey began when she experienced severe skin allergies and sensitivities caused by conventional beauty products. Frustrated with the lack of safe and gentle options, she decided to take matters into her own hands. Jane extensively researched natural ingredients and worked with experts to develop a line of skincare products that are free from harsh chemicals and artificial additives. Her brand quickly gained popularity, attracting a loyal following of individuals seeking healthier alternatives for their skin.

Another brand at the forefront of the green beauty movement is Green Glow. Their commitment to sustainability goes beyond the ingredients they use. They prioritize eco-friendly packaging, opting for recyclable or biodegradable materials. Green Glow also actively supports ethical sourcing practices, ensuring that their ingredients are obtained from fair-trade and organic suppliers. By promoting transparency and accountability, Green Glow has become a trusted name in the green beauty industry.

The green beauty revolution is not limited to these entrepreneurs and brands alone. Across the globe, countless other innovators are making their mark by creating natural skincare products that cater to a wide range of skin types and concerns. From small-scale artisans to established cosmetic companies, the green beauty movement is gaining momentum and reshaping the way we think about skincare.

Whether you have sensitive skin, are concerned about the environment, or simply want to make healthier choices for yourself, the green beauty revolution offers a world of possibilities. By supporting these entrepreneurs and brands, you are not only taking care of your skin but also contributing to a more sustainable future. Embrace the power of natural skincare and join the green beauty revolution today.

Real-Life Transformations with Natural Skincare

In this subchapter, we delve into the incredible power of natural skincare and how it can bring about real transformations in our lives. Whether you struggle with acne, dry skin, or premature aging, the wonders of natural ingredients can work wonders for your skin, giving you a new lease on life.

Natural skincare is a revolution that has been gaining momentum, and for good reason. The market is flooded with products that contain harmful chemicals and synthetic ingredients that may provide temporary solutions but ultimately harm our skin in the long run. The Green Beauty Revolution is here to change that narrative, showing you how to unleash the power of natural skincare and achieve lasting results.

If you've been battling acne for years, it's time to put an end to the cycle of harsh treatments that only exacerbate the problem. Natural skincare offers a gentler and more effective approach to treating acne. By incorporating ingredients like tea tree oil, witch hazel, and aloe vera into your skincare routine, you can say goodbye to blemishes and hello to clear, radiant skin.

For those struggling with dry skin, natural skincare is a game-changer. Harsh weather conditions, excessive use of chemical-laden products, and even aging can contribute to dryness. However, by nourishing your skin with natural oils like argan oil, jojoba oil, and shea butter, you can restore your skin's natural moisture barrier and achieve a soft, supple complexion.

Premature aging is a concern for many, but natural skincare can help turn back the hands of time. Instead of resorting to invasive procedures or expensive creams, harness the power of natural ingredients like rosehip oil, vitamin C, and green tea extract. These antioxidants and collagen-boosting elements can help reduce the appearance of fine lines and wrinkles, giving you a youthful glow without any harmful side effects.

The Green Beauty Revolution is not just about achieving external transformations; it's about embracing a holistic approach to skincare that promotes overall well-being. When we use natural, organic products on our skin, we are not only enhancing its health but also minimizing our exposure to toxins that can harm our bodies and the environment.

So, whether you're looking to address specific skin concerns or simply want to embark on a journey towards healthier, more radiant skin, natural skincare is your answer. The transformative power of natural ingredients is waiting to be harnessed, and by embracing this revolution, you can unlock a world of beauty and self-care that will leave you feeling rejuvenated and confident.

Celebrity Endorsements and Influencers in the Natural Beauty Space

In recent years, the natural beauty industry has witnessed a significant rise in the use of celebrity endorsements and influencers to promote their products. With the growing awareness and demand for clean, chemical-free skincare, these celebrities and influencers have become powerful advocates for natural beauty brands. This subchapter explores the impact of celebrity endorsements and influencers in the natural beauty space, and how they have influenced the skincare choices of people from all walks of life, particularly those concerned about their skin.

Celebrities have long been associated with beauty and glamour, and their endorsement of natural skincare products adds a sense of credibility and desirability to these brands. When a well-known celebrity, who is known for their flawless skin, endorses a natural beauty brand, it sends a powerful message to their fans and followers. The association with a celebrity can create a sense of trust and reliability in the minds of consumers, making them more inclined to try these products themselves.

Furthermore, influencers, who are individuals with a significant following on social media platforms, have become key players in the natural beauty space. These influencers are often regular people who have built a strong online presence by sharing their skincare routines, product reviews, and personal experiences. Their authenticity and relatability resonate with their followers, who see them as trusted sources of information and inspiration.

The influence of these celebrities and influencers extends beyond just product endorsements. They are also shaping the conversation around natural beauty and encouraging people to embrace their natural skin. By promoting a more holistic and sustainable approach to skincare, they are challenging the conventional beauty standards and encouraging people to prioritize self-care and self-acceptance.

For individuals concerned about their skin, celebrity endorsements and influencers provide a valuable resource for discovering new natural beauty products and learning about effective skincare routines. They offer a platform for sharing personal experiences and recommendations, which can be incredibly helpful in navigating the vast array of options available in the market.

However, it is essential to approach these endorsements and recommendations with a critical eye. While celebrities and influencers may genuinely believe in the products they endorse, it is crucial to do your own research and consider your individual skincare needs before making any purchasing decisions. What works for one person may not necessarily work for another, and it is essential to find what truly suits your skin.

In conclusion, celebrity endorsements and influencers have played a significant role in promoting natural beauty products and influencing skincare choices. Their impact has been far-reaching, appealing to people from all walks of life, particularly those concerned about their skin. However, it is essential to use these endorsements and recommendations as a starting point and make informed decisions based on your individual skincare needs. Ultimately, the power of natural skincare lies in the hands of each individual, and the journey towards healthier, radiant skin begins with understanding and embracing your unique beauty.

Global Initiatives and Organizations Supporting Natural Skincare

In recent years, there has been a significant shift towards natural skincare products, driven by a growing awareness of the harmful chemicals and toxins present in traditional beauty products. This movement has gained momentum, and today we see a number of global initiatives and organizations working tirelessly to promote and support the use of natural skincare.

One such organization is the Environmental Working Group (EWG), a nonprofit organization that focuses on advocating for healthier living. Their Skin Deep database is a valuable resource for consumers, providing them with information on the safety of various skincare and cosmetic products. By rating these products based on their ingredients and potential health risks, the EWG enables individuals to make informed choices and opt for safer alternatives.

Another prominent initiative in the natural skincare arena is the Campaign for Safe Cosmetics. This coalition of over 200 organizations is committed to eliminating harmful chemicals in personal care products and replacing them with safer alternatives. Through public education campaigns, lobbying efforts, and partnerships with businesses, the Campaign for Safe Cosmetics aims to protect consumers from toxic ingredients and ensure the availability of safer skincare options.

Additionally, the Sustainable Cosmetics Summit is an annual event that brings together industry professionals, policymakers, and experts to discuss and promote sustainability in the cosmetics sector. The summit focuses on topics such as green formulations, ethical sourcing, and eco-design, providing a platform for knowledge-sharing and collaboration.

The rise of natural skincare has also spurred the growth of organizations dedicated to supporting fair trade practices and promoting ethical sourcing of ingredients. For instance, the Fairtrade Foundation certifies skincare brands that meet their stringent standards for fair trade, ensuring that farmers and workers receive fair compensation for their labor and that environmental sustainability is prioritized.

Furthermore, there are numerous online communities and platforms that encourage individuals to adopt a more natural approach to skincare. These platforms offer a wealth of information, including DIY recipes, product reviews, and discussions on the benefits of using natural ingredients. They serve as a valuable resource for those looking to transition to a natural skincare routine and provide a supportive community for sharing experiences and knowledge.

In conclusion, the global movement towards natural skincare is gaining momentum, thanks to the efforts of various initiatives and organizations. From advocating for safer products to promoting sustainability and ethical sourcing, these entities are driving positive change in the beauty industry. By supporting and embracing natural skincare practices, individuals can not only improve the health and appearance of their skin but also contribute to a more sustainable and ethical world.

Chapter 9: FAQs and Common Misconceptions about Natural Skincare

Is Natural Skincare Suitable for All Skin Types?

In the quest for healthy and radiant skin, we often come across a multitude of skincare products on the market, each claiming to be the ultimate solution for all skin concerns. However, with the rising awareness about the potential harmful effects of synthetic ingredients found in conventional beauty products, more and more people are turning towards natural skincare.

But the question remains, is natural skincare suitable for all skin types? The answer is a resounding yes!

One of the key advantages of natural skincare is its compatibility with various skin types. Whether you have dry, oily, sensitive, or combination skin, there are natural products that can cater to your unique needs. Natural skincare focuses on utilizing plant-based ingredients that work in harmony with your skin, rather than harsh chemicals that can disrupt its natural balance.

For those with dry skin, natural moisturizers enriched with ingredients like shea butter, jojoba oil, or avocado oil can provide intense hydration without clogging pores. Similarly, individuals with oily skin can benefit from natural products that contain ingredients like tea tree oil or witch hazel, known for their ability to regulate sebum production and minimize breakouts.

Sensitive skin, often prone to redness and irritation, can greatly benefit from gentle natural ingredients such as chamomile, aloe vera, or calendula. These botanical extracts possess soothing properties that can calm and nourish the skin without causing any adverse reactions.

Moreover, natural skincare is not only suitable for different skin types but also addresses a wide range of skin concerns. Whether you are dealing with acne, aging, hyperpigmentation, or uneven texture, there are natural solutions available. Ingredients like green tea, vitamin C, hyaluronic acid, and rosehip oil have been proven to effectively combat these issues, promoting a healthier and more youthful complexion.

It is important to note that just because a product is natural doesn't mean it is automatically suitable for all skin types. It is crucial to read labels, understand your skin's specific needs, and choose products that are formulated with your skin type in mind. Consulting with a skincare professional or dermatologist can also provide valuable insights and guidance in selecting the right natural products for your skin.

In conclusion, natural skincare is indeed suitable for all skin types. By embracing the power of nature and harnessing the benefits of plant-based ingredients, we can achieve healthier, more radiant skin without compromising its natural balance. So, why not join the green beauty revolution and unlock the true potential of natural skincare for your skin's well-being?

Can Natural Skincare Treat Serious Skin Conditions?

When it comes to skincare, many of us are constantly on the lookout for effective and safe solutions to address our skin concerns. Whether it's acne, eczema, psoriasis, or rosacea, serious skin conditions can have a significant impact on our well-being and self-confidence. While conventional treatments often rely on harsh chemicals and synthetic ingredients, the rise of natural skincare has sparked curiosity about its potential to treat these conditions.

The good news is that natural skincare can indeed offer a gentle and effective approach to managing serious skin conditions. By harnessing the power of nature's ingredients, these products can provide relief, nourishment, and support for the skin's natural healing process.

One of the key advantages of natural skincare is its focus on gentle and non-toxic ingredients. Synthetic skincare products often contain harsh chemicals that can aggravate sensitive skin and worsen existing conditions. Natural skincare, on the other hand, utilizes plant-based ingredients like aloe vera, chamomile, tea tree oil, and lavender, which are known for their soothing and calming properties. These ingredients work to reduce inflammation, redness, and irritation, providing relief for conditions such as eczema and rosacea.

Moreover, natural skincare products are often free from common allergens and irritants. Many serious skin conditions are triggered or exacerbated by allergens found in conventional skincare, such as fragrances, preservatives, and artificial colors. By opting for natural alternatives, individuals with sensitive skin can minimize the risk of adverse reactions and find relief from their conditions.

Another benefit of natural skincare is its emphasis on nourishing and hydrating the skin. Dryness is a common symptom of many serious skin conditions, including psoriasis and eczema. Natural ingredients like shea butter, jojoba oil, and coconut oil are rich in essential fatty acids, vitamins, and antioxidants. These nutrients help to restore the skin's moisture barrier, soothe dry patches, and promote overall skin health.

While natural skincare can offer relief and support for serious skin conditions, it's important to note that individual results may vary. Every person's skin is unique, and what works for one individual may not work for another. It's essential to consult with a dermatologist or skincare professional to determine the best course of action for your specific condition.

In conclusion, the power of natural skincare should not be underestimated when it comes to treating serious skin conditions. By opting for gentle, non-toxic ingredients and nourishing the skin with plant-based goodness, individuals can find relief, comfort, and improved skin health. Remember, healthy skin is achievable, even for those dealing with serious skin conditions, through the green beauty revolution.

Debunking Myths: Natural Skincare vs. Traditional Skincare

In the quest for healthy, glowing skin, there has been an ongoing debate between natural skincare and traditional skincare methods. With the rise of the green beauty movement, many myths and misconceptions have emerged surrounding these two approaches. In this subchapter, we aim to debunk these myths and shed light on the benefits and drawbacks of both natural and traditional skincare.

Myth 1: Natural Skincare is Ineffective
One common misconception is that natural skincare products are not as effective as their traditional counterparts. However, this couldn't be further from the truth. Natural skincare harnesses the power of botanical ingredients, such as essential oils, plant extracts, and vitamins, which have been used for centuries to nourish and heal the skin. These ingredients can effectively address various skin concerns, including acne, inflammation, and aging, without the harsh side effects often associated with synthetic chemicals found in traditional skincare.

Myth 2: Traditional Skincare is Always Harmful
While it's true that some traditional skincare products contain potentially harmful ingredients like parabens, sulfates, and synthetic fragrances, it is important to note that not all traditional skincare products are bad for the skin. Many reputable brands have made significant strides in formulating safer and more effective products. The key is to read labels carefully, do your research, and opt for reputable brands that prioritize transparency and use ingredients that are proven to be safe for the skin.

Myth 3: Natural Skincare is Expensive

Another misconception is that natural skincare products are excessively expensive. While it's true that some high-end natural skincare brands can be pricey, there are also many affordable options available. Additionally, natural skincare often focuses on quality ingredients and minimal packaging, which can lead to long-term savings and a reduced environmental impact.

Myth 4: Traditional Skincare is Always Tested on Animals

While animal testing has been prevalent in the beauty industry, many traditional skincare brands have shifted towards cruelty-free practices. It is essential to research brands that align with your values and support those that prioritize ethical and sustainable practices.

Ultimately, the choice between natural and traditional skincare depends on personal preferences, skin type, and individual needs. The key is to educate yourself, understand your skin's unique requirements, and make informed decisions based on reliable information. A combination of both approaches can be the ideal solution, allowing you to enjoy the best of both worlds and achieve healthy, radiant skin.

Addressing Safety Concerns and Regulatory Issues

In the fast-paced world of skincare, it is easy to get swept up in the latest trends and products promising miraculous results. However, ensuring the safety and regulatory compliance of the products we use on our skin is of utmost importance. This subchapter aims to shed light on the safety concerns and regulatory issues surrounding the skincare industry, providing valuable insights to everyone interested in maintaining healthy and radiant skin.

One of the primary safety concerns in skincare revolves around the ingredients used in the products we apply to our skin. Many conventional skincare products contain harmful chemicals that can have adverse effects on our health and the environment. These chemicals, such as parabens, sulfates, and phthalates, have been linked to various health issues, including allergies, hormone disruption, and even cancer. It is crucial for everyone, regardless of their skin type or concerns, to be aware of the potential risks associated with these ingredients.

Regulatory issues also play a significant role in the skincare industry. Different countries have varying regulations and standards when it comes to skincare product formulation and labeling. This can make it challenging for consumers to navigate and make informed choices. However, there are certain certifications and labels to look out for, such as USDA Organic, Ecocert, and Leaping Bunny, which indicate that a product has met specific safety and environmental standards.

To address these safety concerns and navigate the regulatory landscape effectively, it is essential to educate ourselves about the ingredients commonly found in skincare products. Understanding the purpose and potential risks associated with each ingredient empowers us to make informed decisions when purchasing skincare products. Furthermore, opting for natural and organic skincare brands can significantly reduce exposure to harmful chemicals.

In addition to personal responsibility, advocating for stricter regulations and transparency within the skincare industry is crucial. By supporting organizations and campaigns that aim to improve regulations and hold companies accountable for their product claims, we can contribute to a safer and more trustworthy skincare market.

In conclusion, addressing safety concerns and regulatory issues in skincare is vital for everyone, regardless of their skin type or concerns. By being informed about the potential risks associated with certain ingredients and understanding the regulatory landscape, we can make conscious choices to prioritize our skin's health and well-being. Together, we can revolutionize the skincare industry, unleashing the power of natural skincare for a healthier and more sustainable future.

Chapter 10: Embracing the Green Beauty Revolution

Incorporating Natural Skincare into Your Lifestyle

In today's fast-paced world, it's easy to neglect our skin and the importance of maintaining its health. Our skin is not only the largest organ in our bodies, but it also acts as a protective shield against external elements. To truly care for our skin, it's crucial to incorporate natural skincare into our daily routines. By doing so, we can unleash the power of nature and experience the transformative effects it has on our skin.

Natural skincare involves using products made from plant-based ingredients, which are free from harmful chemicals and synthetic additives. These products harness the healing properties of botanical extracts, essential oils, and other natural substances to nourish and rejuvenate the skin. Unlike conventional skincare products, which often contain toxins that can harm our skin and overall well-being, natural skincare is gentle, effective, and safe for all skin types.

One of the primary benefits of incorporating natural skincare into your lifestyle is the ability to address specific skin concerns. Whether you struggle with acne, dryness, sensitivity, or signs of aging, there are natural remedies available to help you achieve healthier, more radiant skin. For instance, tea tree oil is known for its antibacterial properties and can be used to combat acne, while rosehip oil is rich in antioxidants and vitamins that promote skin regeneration and reduce the appearance of fine lines and wrinkles.

Moreover, natural skincare is not just about the products we use but also the rituals we adopt. By embracing a holistic approach to skincare, we can create a serene and mindful environment for ourselves. Taking the time to cleanse, tone, and moisturize our skin can become a self-care ritual that allows us to connect with ourselves on a deeper level. Additionally, incorporating practices like facial massage or using a jade roller can improve circulation, reduce puffiness, and enhance the absorption of skincare products.

Incorporating natural skincare into your lifestyle also extends beyond topical applications. It's essential to nourish your skin from within by making conscious choices about your diet and lifestyle. Consuming a balanced diet rich in fruits, vegetables, and whole grains provides your skin with essential nutrients and antioxidants that promote its health. Additionally, staying hydrated, getting regular exercise, and managing stress levels are all crucial factors in maintaining healthy skin.

In conclusion, incorporating natural skincare into your lifestyle is a transformative journey that benefits not only your skin but also your overall well-being. By choosing products made from natural ingredients, adopting mindful skincare rituals, and nourishing your skin from within, you can unlock the power of nature and experience the true beauty revolution. So, embrace the green beauty movement and let nature work its magic on your skin - you deserve it!

Taking Steps Towards a More Sustainable Beauty Routine

In today's world, where environmental concerns are at the forefront of everyone's minds, it is crucial to consider the impact our beauty routines have on the planet. Taking steps towards a more sustainable beauty routine not only benefits the environment but also promotes healthier skin. By opting for natural skincare products and adopting eco-friendly practices, you can make a positive difference for both your skin and the planet.

One of the first steps towards a more sustainable beauty routine is to educate yourself about the harmful ingredients commonly found in conventional skincare products. Many of these products contain chemicals that not only harm your skin but also pollute water bodies and contribute to the depletion of natural resources. By choosing natural skincare alternatives, you can avoid exposing your skin to these harmful chemicals and reduce your environmental footprint.

When it comes to natural skincare, the market offers a wide range of options. Look for products that are made with organic and sustainably sourced ingredients. These products are not only better for your skin but also promote responsible farming practices and protect biodiversity. Additionally, consider supporting brands that use eco-friendly packaging, such as recyclable or biodegradable materials.

In addition to choosing natural skincare products, you can also adopt sustainable practices in your daily beauty routine. For instance, instead of using disposable makeup wipes, opt for reusable cloths or cotton pads that can be washed and used multiple times. This simple swap not only reduces waste but also saves you money in the long run.

Another effective way to minimize your environmental impact is by conserving water. Turn off the tap while applying skincare products or brushing your teeth, and consider taking shorter showers. By being mindful of your water usage, you can contribute to water conservation efforts and reduce your carbon footprint.

Lastly, consider supporting local and sustainable beauty brands. By purchasing from local producers, you reduce carbon emissions associated with long-distance shipping. Additionally, supporting brands that prioritize sustainability encourages other companies to follow suit, ultimately leading to a more environmentally conscious beauty industry.

Taking steps towards a more sustainable beauty routine is an empowering way to care for your skin while also protecting the planet. By choosing natural skincare products, adopting eco-friendly practices, and supporting sustainable brands, you can make a significant impact on the health of your skin and the environment. Start today and be part of the green beauty revolution!

Spreading Awareness and Inspiring Others

In this subchapter, we delve into the importance of spreading awareness and inspiring others to embrace the power of natural skincare. We believe that everyone, regardless of their background or skin type, can benefit from incorporating green beauty practices into their daily routines.

Skin is the largest organ of the body, serving as a protective barrier against external factors. However, it is also highly absorbent, meaning that what we apply to our skin can have a direct impact on our overall health and well-being. Unfortunately, many conventional skincare products contain harmful chemicals that can disrupt our body's natural balance and potentially lead to long-term health issues.

By spreading awareness about the potential dangers lurking in conventional skincare products, we empower individuals to make informed choices about the products they use on their skin. Through education and highlighting the benefits of natural skincare, we aim to create a ripple effect that encourages others to join the green beauty revolution.

One of the most effective ways to spread awareness is through sharing personal experiences and success stories. By discussing the positive changes we have witnessed in our own skin and overall health after transitioning to natural skincare, we inspire others to take a leap of faith and embark on their own green beauty journey.

Additionally, we encourage readers to become ambassadors for the green beauty movement by sharing their newfound knowledge with friends, family, and even strangers. By engaging in conversations about the importance of natural skincare and recommending high-quality green beauty brands, we collectively contribute to a more sustainable and healthier future.

Furthermore, we emphasize the power of social media and online platforms in reaching a wider audience. Through sharing informative content, product recommendations, and engaging with like-minded individuals, we can inspire and motivate others to make conscious choices when it comes to their skincare routine.

Ultimately, the goal of spreading awareness and inspiring others is to create a shift in the skincare industry and promote the use of safe and effective natural alternatives. Together, we can make a significant impact on our own lives, as well as the health of our planet. Let us unite in the green beauty revolution and unleash the power of natural skincare for a brighter and healthier future.

The Power of Natural Skincare in Transforming Lives

Introduction:

In today's fast-paced world, where stress, pollution, and artificial products surround us, it's no wonder that our skin suffers. However, there is a solution that lies in the hands of nature itself – natural skincare. This subchapter delves into the transformative power of natural skincare and how it has the potential to revolutionize not only our skin but also our lives.

The Skin's Connection to Overall Well-being:

Our skin is the largest organ of our body and plays a crucial role in protecting us from external threats. However, it is not just a barrier; it also reflects our internal health. When our skin is healthy and glowing, it boosts our self-confidence and overall well-being. Natural skincare recognizes this connection and aims to nourish the skin from within.

Harnessing the Power of Nature:

Nature has provided us with an abundance of potent ingredients that have been used for centuries to beautify the skin. From aloe vera's soothing properties to the antioxidants found in green tea, natural skincare products harness the power of these ingredients to heal and rejuvenate the skin. By using natural skincare, we tap into the wisdom of nature, avoiding harmful chemicals and synthetic additives that can cause more harm than good.

Addressing Skin Concerns Naturally:

Natural skincare is not just about maintaining healthy skin; it also addresses various skin concerns such as acne, dryness, and signs of aging. For instance, tea tree oil, known for its antibacterial properties, can help combat acne, while jojoba oil deeply moisturizes the skin without clogging pores. By using these natural remedies, we can achieve healthier and more radiant skin without resorting to harsh chemicals.

Embracing Sustainability:

In addition to benefiting our skin, natural skincare aligns with the principles of sustainability. Many natural skincare brands emphasize eco-friendly practices, using organic and ethically sourced ingredients, and minimizing their carbon footprint. By choosing natural skincare products, we not only care for our skin but also contribute to a greener and cleaner planet.

Conclusion:

The power of natural skincare in transforming lives is undeniable. By embracing natural ingredients and avoiding harmful chemicals, we can achieve healthier, more radiant skin while also promoting sustainable practices. Natural skincare goes beyond external beauty; it nourishes our skin, boosts our self-confidence, and enhances our overall well-being. So, why not embark on a green beauty revolution and experience the transformative power of natural skincare for yourself?

In today's fast-paced and increasingly polluted world, taking care of our skin has become more important than ever. Our skin, being the largest organ of the body, is constantly exposed to harmful environmental factors that can wreak havoc on its health and appearance. That is why the power of natural skincare should not be underestimated.

Natural skincare refers to products that are derived from plant-based ingredients and do not contain any harsh chemicals or synthetic additives. These products work in harmony with our skin, nourishing and protecting it from within, resulting in a radiant and rejuvenated complexion. But beyond the surface-level benefits, natural skincare has the potential to transform lives in ways that extend far beyond mere aesthetics.

One of the most compelling aspects of natural skincare is its gentle yet effective approach to addressing various skin concerns. Unlike conventional skincare products that often rely on harsh ingredients, natural skincare harnesses the power of botanical extracts, essential oils, and other natural elements to heal and restore the skin. This approach ensures that individuals with sensitive skin or specific skin conditions can also benefit from the transformative effects of skincare.

Additionally, natural skincare promotes overall well-being. By choosing products that are free from harmful chemicals, individuals can reduce their exposure to toxins that can be absorbed through the skin and potentially harm their health. This holistic approach to skincare aligns with a growing awareness of the interconnectedness between our skin, body, and the environment.

Moreover, natural skincare encourages sustainability and environmental consciousness. Many natural skincare brands prioritize eco-friendly practices, such as using recyclable packaging and sourcing ingredients from sustainable farms. By supporting these brands, individuals contribute to the preservation of our planet and the protection of its resources.

The power of natural skincare goes beyond the physical benefits; it has the potential to boost our confidence, improve our self-care routines, and foster a deeper connection with ourselves. By investing in natural skincare, we are not only transforming our skin but also embracing a lifestyle that promotes wellness, sustainability, and self-love.

In conclusion, the power of natural skincare is undeniable. By choosing products derived from nature, we can transform our skin, improve our overall well-being, and contribute to a more sustainable future. It is time to unleash the potential of natural skincare and embark on a journey towards healthier, happier, and more radiant skin.

Conclusion: Empowering Yourself with Natural Skincare

In embarking on the journey to write this book, "The Green Beauty Revolution: Unleashing the Power of Natural Skincare," it is essential to express gratitude and acknowledge the numerous contributors and supporters who have made this movement possible. The green beauty revolution is not just a solitary effort, but a collective endeavor that has gained momentum thanks to the dedication and passion of many individuals and organizations.

First and foremost, a heartfelt thank you goes to all the skin enthusiasts who have embraced the green beauty philosophy. Your unwavering support and belief in the power of natural skincare have been the driving force behind this revolution. You have shown that taking care of our skin goes beyond mere aesthetics; it is an essential aspect of self-care that impacts our overall well-being.

We are immensely grateful to the countless experts, scientists, and researchers who have dedicated their lives to studying the powerful properties of natural ingredients. Their tireless efforts have provided us with a wealth of knowledge on the benefits of botanical extracts, essential oils, and other organic substances that rejuvenate and nourish our skin. Their contributions have paved the way for the formulation of safe, effective, and environmentally friendly skincare products.

We also extend our deepest appreciation to the pioneers in the green beauty industry, whose passion for sustainability and ethical practices has inspired countless others to follow suit. These individuals and companies have set a high standard for transparency, cruelty-free practices, and eco-consciousness, driving the industry towards a more responsible and conscious future.

Furthermore, we would like to express our gratitude to the local communities and farmers around the world who cultivate and harvest the natural ingredients used in green beauty products. Their commitment to organic farming and sustainable practices ensures that we have access to high-quality, ethically sourced ingredients that are not only beneficial for our skin but also promote a healthier planet.

Lastly, we would like to acknowledge the readers of this book, as it is your curiosity and eagerness to learn that fuels the green beauty revolution. By choosing to educate yourselves about the importance of natural skincare and making conscious choices, you are actively contributing to the growth of this movement.

In conclusion, the green beauty revolution would not have been possible without the collective efforts of numerous individuals, organizations, and communities. It is our hope that this subchapter serves as a humble recognition and appreciation of all those who have played a part in this transformative journey towards healthier, more sustainable skincare practices. Together, let us continue to unleash the power of natural skincare for the benefit of our skin, our planet, and our well-being.

In embarking on this journey of unveiling the power of natural skincare, it is essential to acknowledge the multitude of individuals and organizations that have played a crucial role in the green beauty revolution. The support and contributions from various stakeholders, including scientists, skincare experts, environmentalists, and passionate consumers, have been instrumental in bringing about a positive change in the beauty industry.

First and foremost, we express our heartfelt gratitude to the skincare experts and scientists who have dedicated their lives to researching and developing effective natural ingredients. Their tireless efforts have paved the way for innovative and sustainable skincare solutions that prioritize the health of our skin and the environment. Their expertise has been invaluable in debunking the myth that natural products are any less potent or effective than their synthetic counterparts.

We also extend our appreciation to the environmentalists and activists who have tirelessly fought for a cleaner and greener planet. Their dedication to raising awareness about the harmful effects of conventional beauty products on our ecosystem has been instrumental in driving the green beauty revolution. By advocating for sustainable practices, they have encouraged both consumers and businesses to adopt environmentally friendly alternatives and reduce their carbon footprint.

Furthermore, we would like to thank the passionate consumers who have embraced the green beauty movement. Your demand for natural and ethical skincare products has sent a clear message to the industry, prompting companies to reformulate their products and adopt more sustainable practices. Your support has been crucial in fueling the growth of the green beauty market and encouraging others to follow suit.

Lastly, we express our gratitude to the organizations and brands that have championed the cause of green beauty. By prioritizing transparency, sustainability, and social responsibility, they have set new standards for the industry. Their commitment to creating products that are safe, effective, and environmentally friendly has propelled the green beauty revolution forward.

In conclusion, the success of the green beauty revolution would not have been possible without the collective efforts of numerous contributors and supporters. It is through their dedication and passion that we have been able to unleash the power of natural skincare. As we move forward, let us continue to recognize and celebrate the individuals and organizations who are driving positive change in the beauty industry, benefiting both our skin and the planet we call home.

Printed in the USA
CPSIA information can be obtained
at www.ICGtesting.com
LVHW022136180524
780462LV00011B/621